EVERYTHIN
KNOW AB(

DR ROBERT YOUNGSON is a Consultant Ophthalmic Surgeon. He studied medicine at Aberdeen
University, and is a member of the Faculty of Ophthal-
mology at the Royal College of Surgeons. He has
published numerous articles on medical topics, and is
also the author of *Everything You Need to know about
Contact Lenses*, *Everything You Need to Know about
Your Eyes*, and *How to Cope with Tinnitus and Hearing
Loss* (all Sheldon Press). He is married, with five
children.

Overcoming Common Problems Series

The ABC of Eating
Coping with anorexia, bulimia and
compulsive eating
JOY MELVILLE

Acne
How it's caused and how to cure it
PAUL VAN RIEL

An A–Z of Alternative Medicine
BRENT Q. HAFEN AND KATHRYN J.
FRANDSEN

Arthritis
Is your suffering really necessary?
DR WILLIAM FOX

Birth Over Thirty
SHEILA KITZINGER

Body Language
How to read others' thoughts by their gestures
ALLAN PEASE

Calm Down
How to cope with frustration and anger
DR PAUL HAUCK

Common Childhood Illnesses
DR PATRICIA GILBERT

Coping with Depression and Elation
DR PATRICK McKEON

Curing Arthritis–The Drug-free Way
MARGARET HILLS

Depression
DR PAUL HAUCK

Divorce and Separation
ANGELA WILLANS

Enjoying Motherhood
DR BRUCE PITT

The Epilepsy Handbook
SHELAGH McGOVERN

Everything You Need to know about Contact Lenses
DR R. M. YOUNGSON

Everything You Need to know about Your Eyes
DR R. M. YOUNGSON

Family First Aid and Emergency Handbook
DR ANDREW STANWAY

Fears and Phobias
What they are and how to overcome them
DR TONY WHITEHEAD

Feverfew
A traditional herbal remedy for migraine and
arthritis
DR STEWART JOHNSON

Fight Your Phobia and Win
DAVID LEWIS

Fit Kit
DAVID LEWIS

Flying Without Fear
TESSA DUCKWORTH AND DAVID
MILLER

Goodbye Backache
DR DAVID IMRIE WITH COLLEEN
DIMSON

Guilt
Why it happens and how to overcome it
DR VERNON COLEMAN

How to Bring Up your Child Successfully
DR PAUL HAUCK

How to Control your Drinking
DRS MILLER AND MUNOZ

How to Cope with Stress
DR PETER TYRER

How to Cope with your Nerves
DR TONY LAKE

Overcoming Common Problem Series

Overcoming Common Problems

EVERYTHING YOU NEED TO KNOW ABOUT SHINGLES

Dr Robert Youngson

MB. CHB., D.O., D.T.M. & H.

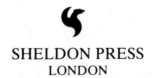

SHELDON PRESS
LONDON

First published in Great Britain in 1986 by
Sheldon Press, SPCK, Marylebone Road, London NW1 4DU

British Library Cataloguing in Publication Data
Youngson, R. M.
    Everything you need to know about shingles.—
(Overcoming common problems)
    1. Herpes zoster
I. Title   II. Series
616.5'22   RC147.H6

ISBN 0–85969–506–9
ISBN 0–85969–507–7 Pbk

Typeset by Deltatype Ltd, Ellesmere Port, Cheshire
Printed in Great Britain by
Richard Clay (The Chaucer Press) Ltd, Bungay, Suffolk

Contents

Introduction

Every year, about four in every thousand people suffer an attack of shingles. The great majority are over fifty years old and the condition gets more and more common with increasing age. It has been estimated that of those who reach the age of eighty-five, half will have suffered at least one attack. And one attack does not confer life-long immunity. Indeed, the likelihood of having a second attack is slightly greater than that of having a first.

Shingles is not a trivial condition, and sometimes the pain which follows it can be severe and enduring. Happily, however, medical scientists have now discovered a great deal about the way in which the virus causing this disease behaves in the body and have developed highly effective ways of dealing with it. We can now identify the people who are especially likely to get shingles. We know what can be done to limit the effects of an initial attack or a recurrence, and how best to manage the complications. In recent years remarkable new drugs have been developed with a quite unprecedented power against the virus which causes shingles – and all stages of the disease can now be treated effectively.

But this new knowledge is not widely available outside the medical profession, and many people, thinking that nothing can be done, experience avoidable suffering. Doctors can now do a great deal for people with shingles, if the help they can afford is sought in the early stages of the condition, when treatment is most effective.

The earliest record of shingles

The first known written reference to shingles was in a manuscript by John de Bartholomeus Trevisa, dated 1398, in which he refers to '. . . icchynge and scabbes wett and drye . . . schingles'. Later entries mention '. . . our Englysshe women call it the fyre of Saynt Anthonye, or chingles'. (The term 'St Anthony's fire' arose from the belief that prayer to St Anthony brought recovery from the 'sacred fire', as the burning neuralgic pain associated with shingles was sometimes called.) The word 'shingles' comes from the Latin 'cingulum' meaning a girdle – appropriate as the distribution of the most common form of the disease is girdle-like. Also, in ancient Greece, the fighting soldier called his belt a zoster. Today, the medical name for shingles is 'herpes zoster'. This should not, however, be confused with 'herpes simplex' – the condition which most commonly takes the form of cold sores round the mouth, or with venereal herpes, although herpes zoster and herpes simplex *are* physically very much alike and can sometimes be treated with the same drugs.

For those who would like to know a little more about the development of our present knowledge of, and treatment of, the condition, I give below a brief medical history. If, however, you prefer to skip this information, please do go on to the first chapter.

Edward Jenner

In the late 1760s, when Edward Jenner was a young apprentice surgeon near Bristol, a young milk-maid came to consult his master on a medical matter. Small-pox having been mentioned, Jenner heard her say, 'I cannot take that disease, for I have had cow-pox.' Cow-pox was a trivial, passing disorder in which the udders of cows, and the hands of their milk-maids, became affected with small blisters. Jenner was intrigued and his subsequent researches showed that cows were subject to two different blistering conditions, one of which did, indeed, give immunity from smallpox. He was also able to show that this protection was only given if contact was made with the blister at an early stage.

At that time, infectious disease claimed many thousands of lives every year. Smallpox, especially, was feared, for the condition was very common, mortality high and those who survived were usually disfigured for life. Jenner pondered upon this problem for thirty years, until in 1796 he came across a milk-maid with cow-pox blisters on her hands, took some of the fluid from them and injected it into a young boy. The boy developed cow-pox with no ill-effects. Two months later, Jenner injected the boy with virulent smallpox from a very ill patient. Had the boy died, Jenner would have faced criminal charges, but, again, the boy showed no ill effects. It was two years before Jenner again found another person with early, active cow-pox, but when he did, he repeated the experiment – with equally satisfactory results. He then published an account of what he had done and soon the correctness of his views were acknowledged by many leading members of the medical profession. He became known the world over and honours were showered upon him.

The Latin for a cow is 'vacca' and the virus we now call 'vaccinia' is a strain similar to the one used by Jenner. The method of transmitting the virus to other people, for the purpose of protecting them against smallpox, was therefore called 'vaccination'. Smallpox has, quite recently, now been eradicated, thanks largely to Jenner. He also started something which has had a much wider effect than simply the control, and eventual eradication, of that disease.

Louis Pasteur

Jenner's success with cow-pox was based on observation and experiment and he did not have the least idea of how it worked. More than fifty years were to pass before we even began to understand how infectious disease was transmitted from one person to another and this was achieved by a young French chemist named Louis Pasteur.

Pasteur's most important work was undertaken as a result of a suggestion made to him for purely commercial motives. The French wine industry was losing millions of francs each year because so much wine, instead of maturing, was turning to vinegar. In 1856, the 30-year-old Pasteur was asked to tackle this problem. When he examined samples of wine under the microscope, he spotted that the yeast cells in good wine were spherical and those in sour wine were elongated. His further research showed that one kind broke down sugar to alcohol while the other produced acetic acid (vinegar). Also, all the yeast left in the wine could be destroyed if the wine were heated to about 50 degrees centigrade and thereby prevent souring. This simple process came to be known as 'pasteurization' and milk has been treated in this way ever since.

Pasteur then set out to discover whether the spoiling of meat was caused in a similar way. First he confirmed that meat which had been boiled and at once sealed, did not decay. Then, in 1860, he boiled some meat extract in a flask with a long, narrow, sharply-bent neck. The contents were open to the air but any particles entering the neck settled at the bend and did not get into the flask. Again the meat remained unspoiled.

Pasteur began to feel that human diseases must be spread by some kind of tiny, invisible particles and he proposed the 'germ' theory of infectious disease. In 1865 he saved the French silk-worm industry from failure by finding the parasite that was killing the worms. By then, his reputation was so great that when he recommended that surgeons should boil their instruments and sterilize their dressings, they complied. The results were startlingly successful. Patients undergoing surgery no longer had to suffer the previous inevitable infection.

Pasteur next tackled the deadly disease anthrax. He isolated the organisms responsible, heated them until they were altered, but still alive, and showed that the modified strain could protect animals without causing the disease.

Pasteur next produced a vaccine against rabies, prior to which, rabies had invariably been fatal. The vaccine worked and soon after, the Pasteur Institute was set up in Paris to treat rabies.

Pasteur was not able to see the germs of rabies with his microscope but was still convinced that they were there, though too small to be seen. In this he was correct. The rabies virus is about the same size as the herpes virus with which we are here concerned – about one fifth the size of the smallest body visible by ordinary light microscopy.

Beijerinck and von Behring

In the meantime – just at the turn of the century – a Dutch botanist, Martinus Beijerinck, demonstrated that 'tobacco mosaic disease' could be transmitted to other plants by something in the juice of squashed-up leaves. Beijerinck also showed that infected plants could pass the disease on to other plants, that the juice was conveying something that was alive and could reproduce.

In 1890, a German bacteriologist, Emil Adolf von

Behring was studying tetanus ('lockjaw') and showed that if he took some of the blood serum from an animal with tetanus, and injected it into another animal, the second animal became immune to the disease. He also proved that serum from the immunized animal could confer at least a temporary immunity on a third animal. He went on to tackle the then deadly disease of diphtheria in the same way and produced an 'antitoxin' which, in 1901, won him the Nobel prize.

Landsteiner and the blood groups

Up to this time very little could be done to help people who had suffered severe loss of blood. Attempts had been made to replace that lost with blood from an animal, or another person. In most cases, the transfused blood apparently killed the patient and the practice was therefore widely condemned. But, in 1900, an Austrian doctor called Landsteiner discovered that blood serum (the liquid part) contains an agent which, when mixed with the red corpuscles of other people's blood, will usually cause them to clump together and become useless. Only when this did not happen could the bloods safely be mixed. By 1902 he had shown that there were four 'blood groups' and that if blood of the same group as that of the patient was used, transfusion was safe. When incompatible bloods were mixed, the serum of one attacked the red cells of the other.

Our present understanding of conditions such as herpes zoster would never have been possible without the pioneering work of these men.

1

What is Shingles?

It is not quite correct to call shingles an infection because, although the condition is caused by a virus, this is not, as in other infectious diseases, acquired shortly before the signs of the disease appear. Shingles is caused by the same virus that causes chicken-pox and often seems to come on for no particular reason. But when people think back, they often realise that some significant event occurred shortly before the onset. This may have been another illness, an injury – sometimes to the part in which the rash later appeared – or a stressful event of some kind, even one apparently unconnected with the body. Stress causes the release of cortisol – a hormone which can interfere with the immune mechanisms of the body, and the activation of the shingles virus is connected with these mechanisms.

The first indication that you have shingles may be a slight fever, a headache, some nausea and a general feeling of being unwell. But the condition usually starts with pain, often occurring in one half of the chest wall in a fairly narrow strip from a point near the spine round towards the front. Alternatively, the condition may affect your face, commonly involving the eyelids and the forehead. Again, it nearly always affects one side only so that the skin rash stops abruptly at the mid-line, and runs up one half of the forehead only. These characteristic areas of distribution correspond to areas of the skin supplied by particular sensory nerves.

Sensory nerves enable us to feel touch, pressure, pain and temperature. They start in the skin (and in muscles, joints and other organs) as 'sensory receptors' – specialized nerve-endings, each type responding only to one particular kind of sensation. So there are specific receptors for touch or pressure, or pain or whatever the stimulus may be. The entire surface of the skin is covered by these nerve endings. With the exception of the face and the front half of the scalp, all the sensory nerves of the body run round to the centre of the back, where they enter the spinal chord and pass up, through it, to the brain. Thus, a constant flow of sensory information keeps our brains aware of our immediate environment so that we are able to avoid extremes of heat or cold or severe pressure or any painful influence which might be an indication that we are in danger.

Occasionally, shingles affect some of the nerves which bring about movement – the motor nerves – but this is fairly rare.

All the sensory nerves are paired on either side of the mid-line of the body so that no one nerve supplies both sides simultaneously. Because the virus tends to affect only one nerve at a time, shingles usually occurs on one side only. However, very occasionally, both members of a pair of nerves are affected, causing the unusual occurrence of shingles on both sides of the body.

The pain of shingles may be constant or intermittent and in the very early stages, it is often mistaken for a symptom of some other disease. Because of the common involvement of the side of the chest (in two people out of three), many patients with early shingles have been thought to have pleurisy (inflammation of the lining of the lung) but, two or three days later, the typical rash appears. In fact, such a mistake should seldom be made as the stabbing pain of pleurisy characteristically occurs on taking a deep breath and is different from that of shingles. Sometimes, if the nerve affected is lower in the trunk, early shingles is mistaken for appendicitis or inflammation in the gall-bladder (cholecystitis) and this is more excusable as the pain may be deep and severe and the early stages are quite often associated with abdominal upset.

The pain can be very variable. Sometimes it is no more than a mild itching or tickling sensation or may not be present at all. During the four or five days before the appearance of the rash, the area of skin involved is often tender to pressure. A valuable early indication of the diagnosis is excessive sensitivity in the affected strip of skin (hyperaesthesia), so that the most gentle touch causes a strong, almost painful, sensation. Many people are familiar with something very similar that happens in the early stages of 'cold sores' developing around the mouth or nose. (Cold sores are caused by a very similar virus, the herpes simplex virus, and the two conditions have a good deal in common). If examination shows that the excessive sensitivity follows exactly the course of supply of one of the spinal or facial sensory nerves, then the diagnosis is almost certain. During this preliminary period, the viruses are active and the person concerned usually has some fever and feels ill.

The rash

About five days after the first sign of the disease the rash appears in the affected area of skin, starting as small, slightly raised, red spots which very quickly turn to tense blisters full of a clear fluid which is teeming with viruses. After about three days the fluid in the little blisters – called 'vesicles' – turns yellowish and, usually within a few days, the fluid disappears, the vesicles flatten, and crusts develop. Over the next two weeks or so these crusts normally drop off, frequently leaving small, pitted scars. Sometimes, the rash can be more severe, with vesicles joining up to form large areas. In such circumstances, healing may take many weeks. In the case of facial herpes there may be some distortion of tissues and loss of normal skin colour.

'Post-herpetic' pain

'Post-herpetic' just means 'after the rash'. Usually, within two or three weeks from the onset, the pain and discomfort will have gone, but in about 30 per cent of people over the age of forty the pain persists for months or even years. The older the person concerned, and the more severe the pre-rash pain, the more likely it is that this will happen. If the rash has been very pronounced, there is also a greater likelihood of prolonged 'post-herpetic' pain. This pain is caused by damage to the sensory nerves so that strong nerve impulses are constantly being produced and passed inward to the brain. The damage will almost always eventually resolve, but this may take months or even years.

Shingles of the face

In 10 to 15 per cent of cases, shingles affects the face. On the whole, facial shingles also tends to be more severe than shingles on the body and there are more complications. The sensory nerve supply to the face, forehead and the front part of the scalp comes from a pair of cranial nerves which emerge directly from the brain, and are called the 'trigeminal' nerves because each of them has three large divisions. The lowest of the three divisions supplies the skin of the jaw, the teeth and the tongue. The middle division supplies the part of the face between the upper lip and teeth and the lower eyelids but not the skin of the nose. From the lower lids up to the highest point of the head and including the eyes, is the first division and it is this one, known as the 'ophthalmic' branch, that is most commonly affected by shingles. Each ophthalmic nerve is confined to its own side of the face and stops at the mid-line. Each carries sensation from the lower lid margin, the skin of the nose on its own side, the cornea of the eye and the eyeball generally, the whole of the upper lid, the eyebrow skin, the forehead and the front half of the scalp. So in ophthalmic shingles we may expect the rash to occupy this area. And if the rash affects the nose, the eye is also likely to be affected. You will find more about this in Chapter 5.

Generalized shingles

This, fortunately, is rare. Generalized shingles may superficially resemble chicken-pox. In any condition in which viruses are spread via the bloodstream throughout the body, there is a possibility that widespread effects may arise but this does not commonly occur in shingles. However, when there *are* less than the usual restraints on the damaging effects of the viruses, trouble may arise from widespread involvement of the nervous system, especially the brain. There may be a generalized inflammation with headache, fits and coma, or, effects very similar to a 'stroke' (cerebral haemorrhage or thrombosis). There may be a paralysis down one side of the body, loss of one half of the field of vision, loss of full control of the eye movements so that double vision occurs and other effects. I would emphasize that these misfortunes are very rare, and that the long-term outcome is usually complete recovery. I mention them solely to reassure those who may have developed them and may be unnecessarily distressed at the prospect of permanent disablement.

Shingles and the nervous system

To understand shingles more fully, it is helpful to have a little knowledge of the nervous system. A nerve cell is but one of many different types of cells of which our bodies are made up. The nerve cell consists of an enlarged part, the body, which contains a central 'nucleus', and one very long nerve fibre. Nerve cell bodies are much too small to be seen with the naked eye, but a nerve fibre may be long enough to reach from the back-bone to the finger-tips. The cell body may lie very near one end of the nerve fibre, which may extend only a little way beyond the cell body. Or the cell body may lie in the centre of a very long fibre – as is the case in most sensory nerves. Major nerves, such as the spinal nerves, are made up of thousands of these nerve fibres, lying parallel to each other.

The nervous system, outside of the brain, has two main sections – the sensory system, which carries information to the brain, and the motor system, which sends out orders to the muscles and enables us to move about. From the under side of the brain a thick column of nerve tissue, called the 'brain-stem' passes down through a large circular hole in the base of the skull, and becomes the spinal cord. This is distinct from the spine, which consists of a series of bones, or vertebrae, graduated in size and each separated from its neighbour by a shock-absorbing disc. Just behind the main mass of each vertebra is an oval hole, and because the vertebrae are set one on top of the other, these holes form a tube through which runs the spinal cord.

The vertebrae lock into each other and are also held in position by strong ligaments. Between each pair of vertebrae there are exit channels for the thirty-one pairs of spinal nerves, each consisting of a quite separate motor and sensory part. The motor nerve connections run down from the brain and the sensory nerve fibres run up to the brain.

At the point at which the sensory nerve fibres pass between the vertebrae, each forms a swelling called a ganglion, where all the nerve cell bodies are found. The ganglion is a sort of junction-box, between the sensory nerve fibres coming from the nerve-endings and those fibres, of the same nerve cells, which pass up the cord to the brain. We have thirty-one pairs of these sensory ganglia, which are very important in shingles, as we shall see. In the case of the sensory nerves for the face, the fibres of each also run into, and out of, a ganglion. This too, has a very important role in shingles, which is a virus infection of the sensory ganglia.

Shingles is caused by millions of viruses which have invaded and damaged one particular sensory ganglion – either spinal or facial. Because the ganglion is the collection of nerve cell bodies and the nerve fibres are continuous with these, when conditions allow, the tiny viruses can move from the cell body in the ganglion, along the fluid in the fibre to reach the nerve ending in the skin and cause the rash.

What is a virus?

The original meaning of the word 'virus' was 'a poison', but we now use this term for a class of organisms which are so small that they cannot be seen with an ordinary light microscope. To see them, we have to use a more powerful instrument called an electron microscope.

The virus we are concerned with, here, is called the 'varicella-zoster' virus. Its total diameter is about one fifth of a micron – and a micron is a mere one millionth of a metre. So it is a small creature to be such a nasty piece of work. 'Varicella-zoster' is a bit of a mouthful, and as I shall have to refer to it frequently, I shall call it 'VZ'.

It lives only a few hours outside the body and it is quite easy to disinfect contaminated materials. When VZ virus is grown in a tissue culture (living cells kept alive in a laboratory) it causes exactly the same kind of damage as it does in the cells of the body.

Electron microscopic examination of the VZ virus shows that it contains a central core of DNA (deoxy-ribonucleic acid), the blueprint for the manufacture of new cells. DNA is made up of genes and these are individual instructions by which protein, the main building material of cells, is reproduced. Viruses also carry their own plans, but – unlike normal cells – they do not have the materials to do the work of reproduction, so they are totally dependent on people's body cells for their survival. As soon as they are inside the host cell, the DNA cores of the viruses replicate in the manner of DNA anywhere and the new viruses then migrate out through the cell membranes, into other host cells. If the virus population within a cell becomes too large, the cell gets overcrowded and often it is killed.

Now different viruses have special preferences for the kind of properties they want to occupy and the VZ virus feels most at home in nerve cells. It is the activity of the virus living within the cell body, and the fibre running from the cell body to the nerve-ending, that causes all the trouble.

2

Chicken-pox and Shingles

We have seen that both chicken-pox and shingles are caused by the varicella-zoster virus, but these two conditions are fundamentally different in their nature and in their effect upon people. Chicken-pox is, almost always, a trivial condition – a passing and usually minor event of childhood – whereas shingles is distressing, and can be serious. So wherein lies the difference? Before this question can be answered we must look at those features which the two diseases have in common.

Most of the common facts about chicken-pox are well known. It usually catches children between the ages of two and eight years, especially when they go to school, and can then spread round the family like wildfire. Chicken-pox is, however, essentially a disease of childhood and tends to be a fairly mild affair. Most children experience relatively little upset, but in very young babies and in older people, it can be quite severe. The virus can even pass through the placenta to infect the unborn baby and in consequence babies have been born with a chicken-pox rash. Happily, in such a case, the disease is usually prevented from being too serious by protective antibodies, which come from the mother and attack the viruses. Very rarely, if a pregnant woman gets chicken-pox during the first few weeks of pregnancy, the foetus may be infected with VZ viruses and consequently have congenital abnormalities. But the risk of this happening *is* very small.

Susceptible people can pick up chicken-pox from a person with shingles, but it is very uncommon for shingles to develop as a result of exposure to chicken-pox. Chicken-pox is commonest in the winter and spring and tends to occur in large epidemics every three years or so. Between epidemics there are few cases. Shingles is hardly infectious at all and shows neither a seasonal pattern nor any relationship to the chicken-pox epidemics. In fact, there is definite evidence that shingles is *less* common during a chicken-pox epidemic. We will come back to this later.

Chicken-pox can be passed on even before the rash appears, probably during the whole of the day before the spots come out; and the patient continues to be infectious until all the tiny blisters have dried out and crusted. The disease is spread by breathing in virus-infected droplets coughed out by a patient. In addition it can be acquired by direct contact. The blisters teem with VZ virus and the disease can also be passed on to someone else by contamination of any object coming in contact with them. Such contamination is infective, however, only for a few hours because the virus cannot live very long outside the body.

Clinical signs of chicken-pox

The 'incubation period' of any infectious disease is the length of time between picking up the infection and the first appearance of the disease. In chicken-pox this varies from about ten days to three weeks, but is usually about two weeks. A day or two before the rash appears, there may be slight fever and a feeling of sickness. Sometimes there is headache and muscle ache. The rash starts as tiny, flat red spots but these progress very rapidly through the stages of clear vesicles, milky vesicles, crusts and scabs. The whole sequence, from red spot to scab, takes only twelve to twenty-four hours and the spots occur in successive crops over a period of from one to six days. Because of this, different spots are often at different stages of development.

The chicken-pox rash does not occur only on the skin. In the very early stages of the disease, tiny blisters develop in the mouth or throat and these ulcerate to provide the source of infecting viruses. Blisters can even form on the membrane covering the whites of the eyes (the conjunctiva), where they do not form crusts, but progress to shallow ulcers which may be quite painful, but usually heal well.

The most serious complication of chicken-pox is encephalitis (inflammation of the brain) and this fortunately is very rare. It is commoner in children than in adults. But only a handful of cases occur each year in this country – and recent developments in treatment of VZ virus infections have provided us with an effective weapon against it.

Infectivity

Chicken-pox is one of the most highly infectious of all diseases, but the commonly held belief – that it is the blisters or the crusts that transmit the infection – is wrong. Indeed tests have shown that it is very difficult to grow VZ virus from chicken-pox crusts. The virus can be obtained from fluid in the blisters and it has been shown that such fluids may remain infectious after freezing at −65 degrees for as long as eight years. But by the time the crusts have dried up there is unlikely to be any live virus left. So elaborate disinfection is quite unnecessary.

The real reason for the infectivity of chicken-pox is that, in the early stages, the child has shallow herpetic ulcers in the mouth and throat which actively shed viruses and these contaminate the saliva droplets in the expired air. So coughs and sneezes, during that period, really spread the VZ viruses and if projected droplets are inhaled by other children, infection is almost inevitable. In the first two or three days, the vesicles, too, are infectious, or rather, 'contagious' and the disease may spread in this way between children playing together.

When infected droplets are inhaled, the VZ viruses are quickly absorbed into the body and spread around everywhere. They have no difficulty in getting through the linings of the lung air-sacs into the bloodstream and are soon scattered throughout the body. Many settle in the skin of the face and the trunk and it is characteristic of chicken-pox that the rash occurs mainly there. But now, a most important thing happens. When the blisters have crusted and flaked off there are still plenty of viruses lying around but these are no longer so active as before. So, instead of just producing more skin blisters, they start looking around for somewhere suitable to squat in peace. As we have seen, they have a preference for nerve cells. And as the quickest route to a nerve cell is by way of a sensory nerve fibre, they make their way up the nerve fibres until they reach the sensory ganglia and there settle quietly, waiting.

This happens in the sensory nerves of the face as well as of the trunk. If, much later in life, shingles occurs, either on the trunk or on the face, the position of the shingles will correspond with the position in which, many years before, the chicken-pox rash was most severe.

So now we move on from the stage at which VZ squatters may settle in and take a look at what happens some forty or more years on, when these viruses again begin to make their presence felt.

The chicken-pox/shingles connection

We have seen how the VZ virus gets into the sensory ganglia. Now we shall see what happens to these viruses when the person concerned later develops shingles. In Chapter 4 I shall deal with the reasons *why* the viruses begin to bestir themselves. Here, we will simply assume that they have come out of their dormant state, in the sensory ganglion and begun to multiply. When they do so, the ganglion becomes intensely inflamed (we call this ganglionitis) and this inflammation causes strong stimulation of the sensory nerves. The brain therefore receives powerful messages that something painful is happening. And because the affected nerve is responsible only for notifying the brain of stimuli coming from its own area of skin, that is where the pain will seem to be coming from.

Examination of ganglia, at this stage, has shown such severe inflammation that some nerve cells are destroyed. It *may* also induce bleeding into the ganglion. The inflammation can sometimes spread to surrounding tissues so that, at the height of the illness, the membranes lining the spinal cord may be affected or, in the case of facial infection, the brain. (This is called meningitis – the linings are 'meninges'.) Ganglionitis, with its resultant powerful stimulation of the sensory pathways to the brain, is the chief cause of any prolonged pain in shingles.

In addition to causing the ganglionitis, the viruses pass down inside the hollow nerve fibres to reach the skin. There they continue to multiply and provoke a local inflammation. The cells in the deeper parts of the outermost layer of the skin degenerate, and become ballooned out by the inflammatory fluid, forming the typical blisters. As in chicken-pox, the blisters teem with

19

viruses. The spread of the virus is much less general in shingles than in chicken-pox, but the severity of the inflammation, where it does occur, is much greater.

Chicken-pox in children

If we could avoid the primary infection, we wouldn't get shingles. But chicken-pox is one of the most infectious of all diseases and it is very difficult for a child to avoid it. If a child who has not had chicken-pox enters a household where there are cases, there is about a 90 per cent chance that he or she will be infected. Very few children avoid it and many suffer the disease without even being aware of it. Lifelong immunity to chicken-pox usually follows an attack.

But there is another, better reason for not trying to prevent children from getting the disease. The condition is nearly always mild in childhood, but this is not the case if it is acquired for the first time in adult life – many complications tend to occur which are very rare in childhood infection. For instance, up to one third of adults who get chicken-pox develop a persistent form of pneumonia which may be severe. The virus may also involve the brain, causing a condition called encephalitis, but this is very rare. Women who get chicken-pox during the early months of pregnancy may sometimes give birth to a baby with congenital malformations. Fortunately, this, too, is very rare.

There is one other reason for not trying to avoid chicken-pox in childhood. Evidence suggests that exposure of adults to chicken-pox virus can protect against shingles, and if it is indeed so we might actually increase the number of cases of shingles if we were to succeed in preventing many children from contracting chicken-pox.

Chicken-pox in adults

This is quite uncommon, but chicken-pox in adults is usually considerably more severe than in children, and is nearly always preceded by two or three days of high fever, shivering, severe headache and backache, cough, sore throat and even breathlessness. The symptoms may suggest pneumonia. When the rash appears, it tends to be widespread and heavy, in proportion to the severity of the previous symptoms. But once the rash is well developed, the adult patient usually feels much better.

A true pneumonia, caused by the VZ virus, is rare but it is always serious. On the second or third day, there is pain in the chest, cough, severe breathlessness with blueness of the skin and a coughing up of blood-stained sputum. In the past, little could be done for patients with severe VZ pneumonia. However, the position is now very much improved.

3

Shingles and Immunity

Today, immunology is one of the most complex branches of medicine and our knowledge is growing so fast that no sooner is a new textbook published than it is out of date. The advances, in the last twenty years or so, have brought into being what almost amounts to a new science and the benefits to medicine – and to people – have been incalculable. Very little of what is now common knowledge was available to us when I was a medical student.

Because the study of immunity has been able to explain and account for a great deal that was formerly confusing and mysterious, I will now give you an outline of some of the basic principles of immunology.

'Self' and 'non-self'

If we take a piece of skin, or indeed any tissue, from one part of a person's body and implant it in some other part – like transplanting a big toe to make a new thumb – there will be no rejection problems and healing will be excellent. As distinct from the problems of implanting 'foreign' tissue, such 'autografts' are nearly always successful unless the purely surgical problems of securing an adequate blood supply prove too great. So it seems that the body has the power of recognizing 'self' and 'non-self' and that it resents the presence of foreign tissue and does what it can to get rid of it – it is, if you like, an allergic reaction.

When we come to the effects of shingles on the eye, in Chapter 5, you will learn that corneal grafting is likely to fail if the cornea receiving the graft is so badly damaged by shingles that new blood vessels have grown into it. Corneal grafting is normally one of the most successful of all grafting procedures, but the presence of blood vessels makes all the difference. The donor disc of clear cornea is taken from the healthy eye of someone who has died and, consequently, is tissue foreign to the person receiving the graft. Under normal conditions, because the host cornea is free of blood vessels, this disc of foreign tissue is effectively isolated from direct contact with the blood of the host. Thus, it seems, the host is prevented from discovering that the tissue is foreign.

The case is very different when foreign tissue which requires a blood supply comes into contact with the proposed host. When early attempts were made to graft human organs, such as kidneys, an angry dilatation of blood vessels occurred within the grafted organ and soon, the whole tissue became intensely inflamed. In almost every case the graft died. Microscopic examination of the rejected grafts showed that their tissues were crowded with millions of white cells. Some of the larger ones were actually taking small particles of the foreign tissue into their bodies, bit by bit. These large white cells are called 'phagocytes'. But for every phagocyte there are thousands of much smaller round cells called 'lymphocytes'.

The 'lymphatic' system is a tissue drainage system in the body, made up of tubes with valves which direct surplus fluid back into the blood stream, after the fluid has passed through 'filters' called lymph nodes, in which the small white cells normally live. There are large collections of lymph nodes in the groins and armpits but they also occur in many other places in the body. If you get ophthalmic shingles, the lymph node just in front of your ear, on the same side, will become painful, tender and enlarged. The lymphocytes normally constitute about 25 per cent of the total white cells of the blood, but increase in number during infection. These small white cells have been more intensively studied than any other cells in the body, because they are vitally important to the whole subject of immunology.

The lymphocytes – basis of immunity

The body resists invasion by any form of foreign material – anthrax germs, shingles or rabies viruses, transplanted tissue, the wrong kind of transfused blood, cancer cells, or whatever – by virtue of one or other of two kinds of lymphocytes. These are the 'B' lymphocytes and the 'T' lymphocytes, cells found in the blood and in the lymph nodes. They are highly mobile, and travel to any site in the body where they are required. They are also very good at reproducing themselves and do so whenever they come in contact with foreign material.

These cells, although apparently all the same, in fact, have a staggering range of subtle variations. This ensures that there will be some lymphocytes naturally suited to attack any particular foreign material. Before starting to reduplicate, the lymphocytes actually select from their numbers those best capable of attacking the enemy. The selected cells then manufacture replicas of themselves. A line of identical cells produced in this way is called 'a clone'.

The 'B' lymphocytes do their job by virtue of substances called antibodies and are mobilized when the body needs to deal with an invasion of large germs, such as the streptococci that cause sore throats, the pneumococci that cause pneumonia and the staphylococci that cause boils. They also act against some viral infections.

The 'T' lymphocytes are most active against viruses, germs which cause long-term, persistent infections such as tuberculosis, infecting fungi, cancer cells and the cells of transplanted foreign tissue.

Protective antibodies

The 'B' lymphocytes all look the same and each one can produce only one kind of antibody, but these antibodies are of almost infinite variety, each capable of dealing with one particular kind of pattern on the surface of an enemy cell. It is by recognizing these surface patterns that the body distinguishes 'friend' from 'foe'. When a few 'B' cells appropriate to the attacker have been selected, each produces a clone of descendants called 'plasma cells' which actually manufacture the antibody molecules within themselves. These protein molecules (called 'immunoglobulins') shoot out at the rate of about 2,000 per second, and lock on to the outer surface of the enemy cells, killing them.

All this takes a few days to develop, so antibodies are not immediately available to combat new infections. But re-infections will induce a strong antibody response. What happens is something like this. Along comes a group of enemy cells, perhaps a few VZ viruses which burst out of nerve cells. The 'B' lymphocytes are chemically attracted to them and immediately begin to feel the surfaces of the viruses. Those 'B' cells that produce an immunoglobulin of the right shape to fit the surface of the enemy viruses are then selected as the defenders. A few of these 'B' cells clone to produce millions of identical, plasma cells and these shoot out immunoglobulins, attacking the viruses with them. The outcome depends on the strengths of the opposing forces. The number of viruses may be temporarily overwhelming so that cellular damage may be done before they can be overcome.

The 'T' lymphocytes operate in a different way. Instead of producing antibodies, they modify their own structure in relation to the shape of the attacker cells. They are especially interested in 'own body' cells whose outer surfaces have been altered as a result of virus squatters within. Such surface modification leads certain 'T' cells to consider that they are dealing with 'non-self' cells and attack them. Other 'T' cells ('helper' cells) assist the 'B' cells to produce antibodies. And others ('suppressor' cells), act as regulators – to prevent the attacking 'B' cells from overdoing things. Incidentally, it is the overaction of these 'suppressor' cells that is responsible for the loss of immune capability in AIDS.

The 'T' cells also attract the larger white cells – the phagocytes – to foreign cells so as to promote their destruction and they produce the anti-viral substance known as 'interferon'. The 'T' cells live from five to ten years, but 'B' cells have a much shorter life span.

However, both 'B' cells, with the particular immuno-globulin needed to attack a particular invader, and 'T' cells, with their various specific protective functions, remain available for many years – sometimes for a life-time. This is because, while individual lymphocytes cannot actually live for years, they do reproduce them-selves, thus remaining always available for cloning to deal with a re-appearance of the original enemy. When that happens, within a very short time enormous numbers of tailor-made lymphocytes are ready to get to work. This is why many infectious diseases occur only once in a particular individual. And this is why Edward Jenner's milk-maids were spared the disfiguring effects of small-pox. Their lymphocytes were stimulated by the very similar cow-pox viruses into producing clones of antibody-producing cells, and the antibody fitted the small-pox viruses so accurately that all those getting into the milk-maids' bodies were destroyed before they could do any harm.

Because of cloning, plasma cells with antibody remain indefinitely in the bloodstream and the amount of antibody present can easily be measured. We can also determine with great precision exactly to what kinds of 'enemy' cells the antibody relates. In other words, we can easily find out what infections a person has had, and how strong is their resistance. Antibody levels to VZ virus seem to remain high pretty well throughout life and these certainly do not prevent people from getting shingles. Indeed, most people who get shingles have quite high antibody levels against VZ virus, which leads us to the question of how it comes about that the VZ viruses start to get active again.

Shingles and the lymphocytes

Young people who have never had chicken-pox have no immunity and the virus spreads rapidly throughout the body, infecting the skin in a widespread manner. The presence of the VZ virus prompts a vigorous lymphocyte response and millions of 'B' and 'T' lymphocytes are formed. The vigorous activity of the 'T' cells soon leads to the destruction of many of the viruses and the free viruses have been mopped up by the 'B' cell antibody (immunoglobulins), so there are no more indications of infection. But by then some of the viruses have found their way into nerve cells, where they are out of range of 'B' cell attack and live there for years, apparently causing little harm.

So how are we to account for the late flare-up of VZ virus to cause shingles? The control exercised by 'T' lymphocytes is called 'cell-mediated' immunity and when this declines, the VZ virus flares up. Clearly, this matter of immune deficiency is central to the issue, not only of shingles, but to our general health. So it deserves a chapter to itself.

4

Immune Deficiency

'Immunity' is rather a loose term, used to refer to the way in which we are protected, to varying degrees, from infecting organisms, foreign material generally and body cells which have undergone cancerous change. As we have seen this protection is provided by 'B' cell clone antibody production, and the more complex 'T' cell activity. 'Immune deficiency' simply means a reduction in the proper functioning of either or both of these two defence systems. Reduced efficiency of these systems, or even their total absence, may in rare cases be found at birth, but it is much more common for it to come on later. We call this 'acquired immune deficiency'.

Acquired immune deficiency is very much in the news these days, but AIDS ('acquired immune deficiency syndrome') though particularly nasty, is by no means the first known example of a failure of the immune system. Immune deficiency states are not uncommon, and probably the commonest cause is simply old age. The explanation for this is given below.

The thymus

Lying at the front of the neck and extending a few inches down into the chest is a small, flat, glandular organ called the thymus. This increases in size until the age of about sixteen and then begins to shrink progressively.

The thymus is of the greatest importance for it is the place in which 'T' lymphocytes develop their special faculties, multiply and mature. Without a thymus there could be no 'T' cells and we would be at risk from virus infections, fungus infections, tuberculosis and cancer.

Having reached maximum size after puberty, the thymus begins to shrink and gradually grows smaller and smaller until, in old age, it may be very difficult to find any thymus tissue at all. Now you may think that old people are therefore at risk of running out of 'T' cells altogether. But things are not as black as that. Remember that 'T' cells can live for ten years, and that contact with chicken-pox later in life offers additional protection against shingles. This can only mean that the presence of new viruses prompts the re-cloning of the appropriate 'T' cells to attack the viruses. So we may not have much thymus tissue left in old age to process *new* 'T' cells, but we still have 'T' cells that can clone.

Do we know what factors encourage shrinkage of the thymus? Well, we know that steroids, both in the form of drugs and as the body's natural steroid hormone, cortisol, certainly do this. One of the most potent causes of steroid secretion in the body is stress and it seems to be fairly generally agreed that stress is a cause of cell-mediated immune deficiency. Most doctors would agree that an attack of shingles often follows injury or other illness or, indeed, almost any stressful episode. The same applies to herpes simplex, the other common herpes virus that causes cold sores (HSV 1) or venereal herpes (HSV 11). The herpes simplex virus behaves in a very similar way to the VZ virus and recurrences of herpes simplex attacks, of both kinds, are often caused by stress.

Shingles and immune deficiency

Doctors talk about certain people being 'immuno-compromised'. This means that their 'B' and/or 'T' cell systems have been damaged or even knocked out altogether. Shingles is very common in people who are immunocompromised for any reason; perhaps, for example, because they have been having large doses of steroids to prevent graft rejection. People should never be given steroids, internally, except for such important reasons, but there are circumstances in which steroids are the only way in which death or serious illness may be prevented. Steroids are by no means the only cause of immunodeficiency. Drugs which interfere with cell division are also a cause. These drugs are used after grafting, in cancer treatment, in rheumatoid arthritis and for other purposes, and patients having them may get shingles because of the depression of the cell-mediated immunity. Prolonged use of antibiotics can also compromise the immune system.

But these are extreme, relatively uncommon cases and the question arises whether the degree of immune deficiency which is the common cause of the reactivation of VZ virus in older people is avoidable. I think that an awareness of the effects of stress and of the other factors leading to immune deficiency may help us to avoid the loss, at an unduly early age, of cell-mediated resistance, not only to infection, but to cancer.

Shingles and the risk of cancer

Let me stress that there is simply no reason at all to suppose that the VZ virus can cause cancer. You may have heard that some viruses have been shown to be the cause of certain cancers. Those viruses that cause cancer in humans and animals are well known and indeed, this is one of the most closely examined areas of cancer research. But there has never been any evidence that the shingles virus is carcinogenic. The result of a major research project into this question was published in 1982 in one of the most respected medical journals. This project involved the follow-up study of 590 people after they had developed shingles. The average follow-up time was nearly sixteen years and, altogether, 9389 person-years were involved in the study. The results showed that the tendency to cancer was exactly the same as in the general population. The authors of this study report concluded that neither special investigation nor long-term follow-up of these people, for cancer, was justified.

This is encouraging for people with a history of shingles, and especially for those who may have heard of the common medical belief that shingles implies a higher cancer risk. But it should be remembered that the conclusion was a statistical one, valid enough as grounds for deciding, as the authors did, that extensive investigation of all such people is unjustified. It should not be taken as a reason, in any one particular case, for not investigating someone who has had shingles and then develops other suspicious symptoms.

Shingles and AIDS

AIDS is now known to be caused by a virus called the 'human "T" cell lymphotropic virus' Type 3, and, because the immune system is effectively turned off by this virus, people with AIDS succumb to infection by organisms which are normally unable to get a foothold in the body. Some die from pneumonia caused by a germ called pneumocystic carinii – a condition practically unknown apart from immune deficiency. Others develop a very rare form of cancer called Kaposi's sarcoma. And, as may be expected, shingles. As we have seen, less than 10 per cent of cases of shingles occur in people below the age of twenty and many of these probably have some immune deficiency. AIDS also is a disease of comparatively young people – the average age is somewhere in the early thirties.

The occurrence of shingles in a comparatively young person with no obvious cause of immunosuppression could therefore indicate the possibility of AIDS. The disease is becoming more common, especially among those with a promiscuous life-style and, although the great majority of those contracting it so far have been homosexual, it is not certain that it is confined to such people. Should the shingles be associated with severe fatigue, weight loss, fever, enlarged lymph glands and raised spots on the skin, then specialist medical advice should be urgently sought.

5

Shingles and the Eye

Shingles varies greatly in its severity, and a mild attack of 'herpes zoster ophthalmicus' (shingles of the face) may be much less troublesome than severe shingles of the trunk. But, in general, shingles affecting the sensory nerve of the face is distressing and disabling. Some people with this condition suffer a constant neuralgia, affecting almost the whole of one side of the forehead and scalp and preventing sleep. The skin too, is sensitive to any contact – even a draught of air. However, the fortunate majority with the fading of the rash, enjoy relief from the pain. And even when this relief does not occur naturally, much can be done nowadays to relieve post-herpetic pain.

The early stages

Ophthalmic zoster usually starts suddenly and with little warning. The person affected feels ill, feverish and unhappy, and is often nauseated. There may also be vomiting. From an early stage there is pain which outlines the skin distribution of the affected nerve. That is, on the side of the bridge of the nose, along the upper eyelid and eyebrow, and up the forehead on the affected side to the topmost point of the head. Sometimes the lower lid is also affected and, occasionally the tip of the nose. As this particular patch of skin is supplied by the same nerve twig that supplies the eyeball, the latter may be at risk. Don't forget to point this out to your doctor, should it happen to you.

The rash

Sometimes the general symptoms, caused by the widespread migration of the viruses, are so severe that the person fails to notice the characteristic distribution of pain in the facial area and the correct diagnosis is not made until the typical rash appears. But this is uncommon. The rash may, occasionally, appear at the same time as the pain but it is usually delayed for three or four days. The first sign is a redness of the skin affecting either the whole or part of the area of distribution of the nerve. The skin may also be markedly swollen and often the temperature of the affected area is well above that of the corresponding skin on the other side. The swelling is especially conspicuous in the upper lid and causes it to droop. But this is, in most cases, simply due to the weight of the fluid collecting in the skin. Should an actual paralysis of the delicate muscle which elevates the lid occur (and this is rare) recovery can usually be expected within about six weeks.

Almost as soon as the redness and swelling occur, the small blisters also appear all over the reddened area. At first they are filled with a clear fluid that very quickly becomes yellow as it fills with VZ virus particles. This fluid is highly infectious to people with low immunity and can easily cause chicken-pox in children. Soon after, the blisters release the fluid, then quickly form scabs.

The pain

From onset to healing of the skin pits, takes from three to six weeks and to the person concerned the worst feature is likely to be, not so much the temporary facial rash, but the neuralgic pain. Remember that we are dealing with an affection of a sensory nerve – a nerve whose sole function is to inform the brain that something is happening to the skin which should be avoided. Pain, in the normal healthy person is a warning to us to do something to avoid whatever it is that is externally stimulating the body in this way. But in the case of a process involving the sensory nerve itself, the messages are being prompted, in a very intense form, by inflammation in the nerve itself.

In a few cases, the pain may be no more than a tingling or numbness. Such people have quite minor involvement of the nerve so that the stimulus sent to the brain is negligible. Regrettably, most people with ophthalmic herpes zoster suffer rather more but, in most cases, the pain settles when the rash heals, leaving only a numbness and tightness in the skin. Finally, there are a few people who continue to experience 'post-herpetic pain' for a long time. This is discussed in Chapter 7.

Involvement of the eye

In about half of those people who contract shingles of the ophthalmic division of the nerve, the disease affects the skin only and they are spared damage to the eye. The other half have eye symptoms which may sometimes last for months. But eye involvement in shingles is usually more an annoyance than an agony – indeed, as I will shortly explain, pain is *not* a common feature.

The early stage is often associated with swelling of the upper lid, which effectively closes the eye and spares the person concerned the temporary mistiness of vision caused by swelling of the outer layer of the cornea. By the time the swelling has gone down vision is usually back to normal and most patients are unaware of what has happened. Because of the swelling, the blisters and the tenderness of the skin during the early stages, examination of the eye is very difficult, even for an eye specialist. But there are ways in which this can be done and this is certainly recommended if, contrary to the common experience, there should be pain which is obviously seated in the eye itself.

Conjunctiva and cornea

Involvement of the conjuntiva is uncommon and not particularly serious. During the active stage, the membrane is inflamed and often swollen and the condition closely resembles any other form of conjunctivitis. Sometimes small blisters similar to those on the skin actually occur in the conjunctiva itself.

Zoster of the cornea is more serious. There is good evidence that VZ viruses get to the cornea along the delicate nerve fibres. One of the effects of the viruses may be to destroy the ability of the hair-fine corneal nerve fibres to conduct impulses. On the one hand this relieves the patient of pain; on the other, it deprives him of any warning of possible damage to the cornea. So foreign bodies, ingrowing lashes, infection and other hazards may cause damage of which the only indication will be blurring of vision.

Whenever the cornea is involved there is always some degree of internal inflammation of the iris (the coloured part) and of the focusing muscle which surrounds it. But often this is mild and passes without ill-effect. It does, however, sometimes happen that the inflammation is more severe and this requires urgent specialist attention if the sight is to be protected. Fortunately, inflammation does not usually start until about a week after the skin rash appears, which gives us time to arrange a specialist appointment. My advice is that every person who develops ophthalmic zoster should once a day check that the vision is normal or only slightly less clear than normal. If this is very difficult to do because of the swelling and tenderness of the lids, I think medical advice should be sought.

Inflammation can lead to a rise in the pressure within the eye as well as adhesions between the iris and the internal lens. This pressure rise is called secondary 'glaucoma' and, if untreated, *may* actually damage the eye so that vision is lost. Drugs such as atropine, corticosteroids and diamox can be used to control these tendencies, but must be used early.

Treatment with drugs which act directly against the viruses can be very effective, but they must reach all parts of the body. This means general anti-viral treatment by injection or, possibly, by mouth. This treatment must be started as early as possible, before damage to the nervous system has been caused. Anti-viral treatment seems to have no place in the treatment of 'post-herpetic' pain and, as you will see in Chapter 7, an entirely different approach is required to this. What we want to do, of course, is so to diminish the intensity of the infection that the attack is mild and the complications absent.

Ideally, of course, shingles should be avoided altogether and it is worth remembering that a boost to one's 'immunity', by exposure to children with chicken-pox, can be useful. A vaccine against VZ virus does exist but, oddly enough, it has little value in the prevention of adult shingles.

Long-term corneal complications

In the majority of cases of ophthalmic shingles, the eyeball itself is not affected. In a small number of people, however, viruses make their way along the fine nerve fibres supplying the eyeball with sensation, and when this happens, specialist attention is required. Most of the eye effects, if carefully managed by the ophthal-mologist, can be controlled, although some can be persistent and difficult.

One such condition results from the loss of the normal corneal sensation because of damage to the nerve fibres. The normal cornea is exquisitely sensitive to touch or to the presence of foreign bodies. This is important for the protection of the corneal surface against injury and ensures that immediate, automatic avoiding action is taken. Even the tiniest particle of grit on the normal cornea leads to the suspension of almost all other action until the irritation is removed. But when the cornea is anaesthetic, as sometimes happens with shingles, this protective reflex has gone, and one may be unaware that damage is being caused.

It is not just grit particles that cause trouble. Because of the anaesthesia, damage to the outer, germ-proof and protective, layer of the cornea may occur, unnoticed. This layer normally has excellent regenerative powers, so that small abrasions (assuming that we keep the eye closed) will quickly heal. But if we are not aware of pain, these abrasions tend to persist and may become infected and turn to ulcers. Should an ulcer occur anywhere within the part of the cornea through which light-rays pass to enter the eye, the vision will be seriously disturbed. So it is very important that specialist treatment begins urgently to avoid such developments.

Shingles and the eye movements

Eye movements are controlled by a delicate mechanism in the stem of the brain with three nerves running, on each side, to the tiny muscles that rotate the eyeballs. These are motor nerves, and fortunately, the VZ virus seems to prefer sensory nerves. Nevertheless, these motor nerves *are* sometimes involved resulting in an interference with the carefully balanced signals going to the eye-moving muscles. On movement, the two eyes no longer necessarily point in the same direction, resulting in uncontrollable double vision – which can be alarming and distressing.

However, I am glad to report that, in the very great majority of cases, the condition recovers spontaneously and completely. Even in those rare cases in which spontaneous recovery does not occur, the condition is by no means irremediable. After some weeks or months, during which the eyes take up a new balance, an operation can be performed to readjust the muscle power so that double vision is abolished or minimized.

Involvement of the tear system

The lacrimal gland (tear-producing gland), which lies just under the bone margin at the upper and outer corner of the eye socket, may be involved in the acute stage of ophthalmic shingles. But this usually goes unnoticed because the lid is so swollen that the inflammatory swelling of the gland is concealed. It is very rare for shingles of the lacrimal gland to cause any permanent harm although, occasionally, the tear flow may be affected.

A more common way in which tear secretion may be interfered with is by involvement of a tiny nerve junction, called the 'ciliary ganglion' which lies within the group of eye-moving muscles, just behind the globe. Involvement of this can cause persistent dryness of the eye, for which ophthalmic treatment will be required. It may be necessary for the affected person to use 'artificial tears' for a long time.

Shingles can also have the opposite effect, producing excessively watery eyes if the tiny ducts which carry the tears away from the eye are scarred following the rash.

So, tear duct blockage can be a most annoying effect of shingles. It may be necessary to insert plastic tubes until a new lining grows round them. Even then, the trouble may recur.

Importance of checking the vision

I recite the above sequence of possibilities simply to make sure that anyone who has had ophthalmic shingles is clearly aware of the importance of seeking medical advice at the earliest indication that anything is wrong. The most important indication is a sudden deterioration in the quality of vision and this should be routinely checked every day. Without becoming obsessive about it, you can, quite easily test the visual clearness of the affected eye:

● It is best to use, as a test object, something in the distance – at least about twenty feet away. Make a note of what one can see – perhaps some writing on a billboard, or something similar – and then, each day, carefully cover up the unaffected eye and check that there has been no change.

● It is also well worth arranging, if one can, for a spouse or a friend to take a look at the cornea of the involved eye, from time to time, using a good light and a magnifying glass. The appearance of any white spots on the surface should be reported to your doctor without delay. Corneal ulceration is not particularly difficult to treat, if spotted early, and ulcers away from the centre of the cornea need not do any permanent harm.

● People who have suffered corneal complications of shingles should be especially careful about using contact lenses. Normally, such contact lenses, especially the hard lenses, are very safe because any major trouble is at once made apparent by pain. But this warning may not be available to people who have had ophthalmic shingles and these must be especially wary. I would advise against contact lenses for people with anaesthetic corneas, because the lenses can cause damage to the outer layer of the cornea. At the very least, such people should be acutely critical of the standard of their vision and should regularly visit a specialist, for the examination of their eyes.

Before ending this chapter, let me remind you that most, if not all, of the developments I have mentioned can be prevented by timely recognition and early treatment. This, of course means early self-diagnosis and no one who has read this book should have the least difficulty in spotting ophthalmic shingles well before the rash appears. As soon as you are aware of any of the warning symptoms, consult your doctor and tell him what you think is wrong. He will probably be impressed and, of course, you will be in a good position to get the treatment you need.

6

Complications of Shingles

The most serious complication of shingles is 'post-herpetic' pain. As we have seen, pain is nearly always present in the early stages of the disease and often goes away some time after the rash appears. But, in about one third of people with shingles, especially those with ophthalmic shingles – the pain continues throughout the active stage of the disease and beyond, persisting for months or even years. Sometimes the pain stops as the rash fades, then, just as recovery seems to be under way, it comes back again and then persists. This 'post herpetic pain' is such an important complication that I have devoted Chapter 7 to it. So I will say no more about it here.

Most of the conditions mentioned below are temporary and respond well to modern drugs, but early treatment is important.

Secondary infection of the rash

Normally, the shingles blisters dry up without complication and heal leaving no trace. But sometimes 'secondary infection' occurs. What do we mean by secondary infection? Well, the healthy skin is remarkably resistant to most germs and effectively keeps out the bugs (staphylococci) that cause pimples and boils. Even in healthy skin, some of these 'staphylococci' occasionally manage to get a toe-hold around the root of a skin hair and cause a boil, but normally, large numbers of them live on the skin surface without doing any harm. A primary infection of the skin with VZ virus, however, lowers the resistance and allows access to secondary invaders such as staphylococci. So the rash becomes infected with pus-forming organisms and the skin in the region of the shingles rash becomes inflamed and may be covered with small pustules.

Such secondary infection may go deep, involving the part of the skin incapable of full regeneration, so that when the skin finally does heal, scarring and distortion may be evident. Tissue distortion is more likely in ophthalmic herpes than in herpes of the trunk. For instance the skin between the upper lid and the eyebrow may form a ridge of scar tissue. Distortions of this sort will sometimes resolve with patience and massage with a skin-softening ointment. If not, the scar tissue can be removed surgically and in some cases minor plastic surgery may be needed.

Tightness around one side of the chest may also be a sequel of secondary infection and scar contracture. Rarely, this, too, may call for plastic correction.

Another possible secondary effect is some local discoloration of the skin. This localized whitening is called 'depigmentation'.

Avoidance, of course, should be aimed for in every case and this means seeking medical advice early. Secondary infection is unlikely if you are having proper medical attention for, at the first sign, effective antibiotics can be given and the tendency checked. You may, perhaps, not be able to get treatment early enough to attack the viruses in the manner described in Chapter 8, but there is no reason why you should not be in time to ensure that the secondary infection is controlled. Nearly all staphylococci are sensitive to one antibiotic or another.

Shingles of the ear

In a shingles infection of the ear, the extent of the involvement can vary considerably. Blisters may form only on the external ear, but often spread into the skin-lined tube leading in to the ear drum and sometimes affect the drum itself or occur further in to involve the middle ear. This not very common form of shingles may be associated with paralysis of some of the muscles on the same side of the face and with loss of the sense of taste in most of the tongue. This odd combination of effects is called the 'Ramsay-Hunt syndrome' after the man who first described it in 1907. It is an example of the fact that the VZ virus, although showing a preference for sensory nerves, will, on occasion interfere with the function of motor nerves responsible for movement. In this case, the one we are concerned with is the motor nerve supplying all the muscles of expression. The Ramsay-Hunt syndrome may cause scarring of the external ear and, if there has been middle ear involvement, perhaps deafness. There may also be disturbance of balance, with vertigo, nausea and vomiting.

Bell's palsy

When one of the motor nerves to the face (there are two – one on each side) is affected by shingles, the face becomes lop-sided, sometimes with drooping of the features on the affected side. The forehead loses its wrinkles on one side and the eyelids may be unable to close. Sometimes the lower lid falls away a little from the eye and this prevents the tears from getting into the tear drainage duct so that they tend to run over. The smile is one-sided and the ability to press the lips together is lost on the affected side.

This condition of facial nerve paralysis has been

known to doctors for a century and a half, as 'Bell's palsy' after Sir Charles Bell, a distinguished Edinburgh surgeon who was the first to make a clear distinction between motor and sensory nerves and to show which were which. In such a case, because the facial nerve is not primarily a sensory nerve, pain will not be a major feature as in the commoner type of shingles. The paralysis will, in many cases, begin to clear up within a few days. About three-quarters of the people affected are back to normal within a few weeks.

Paralysis of the upper eyelid

We have already seen that in the early stages of ophthalmic herpes zoster the upper eyelid is often so swollen with fluid that it hangs down. Once the swelling has resolved, however, the lid position should revert to normal. But sometimes the VZ viruses manage to get into that part of the brain-stem from which the nerve controlling the upper eyelid emerges, and cause a persistent drooping of the lid because the delicate muscle that elevates it is paralysed. This state is called 'blepharoptosis' or, more commonly, just 'ptosis'. Fortunately, spontaneous recovery is usual and, although this nerve also supplies most of the eye muscles, interference with the movements of the eye is very rare.

Sometimes involvement of this nerve has more widespread effects. Another of its functions is to send messages into the eyeball to constrict the pupil. Cases have been recorded in which this function is affected so that the pupil remains larger than the one on the other side. This doesn't however cause the person concerned very much disturbance. More upsetting is the complication in which the power of focusing, of that eye, is affected. The ability automatically to change the focus of the eye when we shift our gaze from near to far objects, is called 'accommodation' and the loss of this faculty, in one eye, is disturbing. Gradual loss of accommodation with age, so that we need progressively stronger reading glasses, is normal and happens to everyone. But the sudden loss of accommodation in one eye is not so easy to accept. Glasses may be necessary for those who are comparatively young when this happens. After the age of about sixty-five there is little or no accommodation to lose, so the condition may pass unnoticed.

I would emphasize that full recovery is possible in all of these motor complications of shingles.

Optic neuritis

This complication of shingles is, again, fortunately quite rare. The optic nerve is probably the most important sensory nerve in the body, for it enables us to see. To be accurate, the optic nerve is not a nerve in the strict sense of the word, but is actually an extension, or tract, of the brain. This is, perhaps, fortunate, for if it were an ordinary sensory nerve, it might be more prone to infection with VZ virus. Nevertheless, the condition does occasionally occur. 'Optic neuritis' simply means 'inflammation of the optic nerve'.

In order to get from the brain to the eyeball, the optic nerve has to pass through a narrow channel in the bone of the skull. The nerve fits tightly into this channel. If VZ viruses somehow get into the optic nerve they may set up a severe inflammation, causing swelling and compression of the nerve and a consequent interference with the ability of the nerve fibres to conduct impulses. This means that the brain will no longer get signals from the retinas and vision will be lost. If the inflammation is very severe, vision will be blotted out completely. But if the inflammation is less severe, vision will be lost only in a central area. This is called a 'scotoma' or 'blind spot' and it is, unfortunately, usually large enough to abolish all useful perception. Central vision enables us to make out detail, read, recognize people, and so on.

Shingles optic neuritis often does not show itself until some considerable time after the onset of the disease. Indeed, many cases have been reported in which the complication has appeared as long as ten weeks after the beginning of the rash. The prospects for restoration of vision are not good. The optic neuritis may damage the nerve fibres so that they cease to function altogether. In spite of this prognosis, recovery *is* possible if specialist care and anti-inflammatory treatment, with steroids, is started soon enough. So, once again, the moral is to seek expert management without delay.

Paralysis of the pupil

This is a much commoner complication than optic neuritis and is much less serious. It often appears months after the shingles attack, and it is almost certainly caused by involvement of the same ciliary ganglion I mentioned in the previous chapter, as a cause of defective tear production. The pupil of the eye, on the same side, becomes widely dilated and thus conspicuously different in size from the other. There will be some loss of clarity of vision and to a varying extent, intolerance to bright light, but spontaneous recovery is possible and drops may be used to constrict the pupil. The affected person will probably prefer to wear sun-glasses in bright conditions, out-of-doors.

Congenital cataract

This complication affects, not the person with shingles,

but her unborn baby. Again, fortunately, it is rare. If a woman develops shingles while she is in the very early months of pregnancy, the VZ viruses can affect the foetus. Because the baby has not yet developed any immunity, the effects can be serious. One of these is the development of cataracts (opaque internal lenses) as a result of interference with the normal growth of the lenses, early in their development. The child will be born blind. A disorder present at the time of birth is known as a 'congenital' condition.

Shingles is, however, quite rare in women of child-bearing age – unless they are immunocompromised. Congenital cataracts can be treated by early surgery and the fitting of special contact lenses, but the condition must be recognized very early. Babies born to women who have had shingles in the first three months of pregnancy should therefore be examined by an ophthalmologist, as soon as they are born.

Paralysis in body shingles

When shingles affects the trunk, the viruses are situated in the ganglion cells of the sensory nerves just where they enter the spinal cord. In this position, the VZ viruses are very close to the corresponding motor nerves, coming out of the cord. It is thus easy to account for the distribution of paralysis when shingles causes this in the muscles of the arms and trunk. For example, a rash on the point of the shoulder may be associated with paralysis of several of the muscles of the arm or hand. Shingles on the neck can be associated with paralysis of the diaphragm and there have even been cases where the viruses have affected the spinal cord itself with resulting anaesthesia of the lower limbs.

Very rarely, shingles affects the buttocks and the

genitals and, when it does so, the urinary bladder is usually involved. This upsets normal bladder function so that passing urine may be very painful. Occasionally it is necessary to insert a plastic tube (a 'catheter') to release the urine.

Shingles and the brain

I want to stress that infection of the brain itself, by VZ viruses, so as to cause either generalized encephalitis (inflammation of the brain) or more local neurological effects, is almost unknown. But as the brain is the centre responsible for producing the initial nerve impulses for all movement, damage to it by VZ viruses *may* cause paralysis. Because one side of the brain produced movement in the other half of the body and because the effect of the viruses tend to be patchy, the usual effect of such motor involvement is a paralysis of one side of the body. If the part of the brain concerned with vision is affected, the result tends to be loss of one half of the field of vision in each eye.

The effects of VZ encephalitis may be very widespread and a wide variety of disturbances of all the functions of the brain – speech, intellect, all the different kinds of sensation and all the delicate bodily control mechanisms – may occur. But, as you will learn in Chapter 8, effective and reliable treatment is now available so that the outlook, even in such a condition, is very much more favourable than it was.

7

Treating 'Post-herpetic' Pain

Persistent pain, situated in the region where the rash occurred, can be a legacy of shingles. Often the pain lasts for several weeks or months, but in an unfortunate few, it becomes permanent. It is to these sufferers that this chapter is especially addressed. Chronic (long-lasting) pain of this kind can have a devastating effect on the life of the unfortunate victim. Many of the people concerned are old and frail and are poorly equipped to handle the resulting serious debility – to say nothing of the deeply demoralizing effects of unremitting and severe pain. Although pain is merely a symptom and does not, under normal circumstances, offer any danger to life, it is no exaggeration to say that proper management of post-herpetic pain, may, in some cases, be life-saving. Without adequate relief, life may become, quite literally, not worth living, and the will to go on living may be lost.

The quality of the pain

The older the patient, the greater is the likelihood of severe post-herpetic pain. If pain has been present for six months, it is likely to be permanent; and it must, unfortunately be accepted that established post-herpetic pain, unless treated, is constant. Relief is obtained only by sleep. Many people with post-herpetic pain report that if they lie perfectly still, on waking in the morning, they can delay the start of the pain. But as soon as they move, it returns. Post-herpetic pain has a peculiar hot quality, and there is sometimes a 'crawling' sensation under the skin. The affected area is commonly extremely sensitive to even the lightest touch. Often firm pressure is more tolerable than light touch and the sufferer may keep a hand tightly pressed, for long periods, to the painful zone. As we shall see later, firm pressure can even relieve the pain a little.

Principles of pain control

Pain is intimately bound up with the state of mind of the sufferer so that, depending on the attitude to it, the same degree of pain may have markedly different significance to the person concerned. Pain associated with fear, for instance – perhaps with fear of disability – is much less tolerable than the same degree of pain experienced by a person confident that it does not imply anything serious. Again, an awareness that the pain will be of limited, or finite, duration enables the sufferer to view it with much more acceptance than if there seems no hope of its remission.

Every doctor is aware of these differences in the attitude of his patients to pain, but not every doctor is aware of how profoundly such psychological factors affect the significance of the pain. Sometimes, if a doctor will take just a few minutes to explain and reassure, this may have the most far-reaching effects on the quality of a patient's life.

So I hope that anyone with post-herpetic pain who is reading this book will derive comfort from having learned that the symptom, however severe, is due solely to the constant stimulation by the virus-induced irritation, of the affected sensory nerves. By the time the post-herpetic pain is established, the active stage of the disease is over and the continuing pain is due to the damage caused during that stage.

However, the depression, and even anger, commonly associated with long-persistent pain may have to be treated by anti-depressant therapy. Anti-depressant drugs do not have any direct effect on pain, but such is the importance of the state of the mind, that these drugs are often very effective in relieving pain. They will usually be employed in conjunction with one or other of the group of drugs known as 'analgesics'. (See below.)

Anger is an understandably common response to prolonged severe pain but anger, as well as being destructive and pointless, uses up valuable energy. It is important for your doctor to be aware of the anger so that he or she can treat it directly.

Importance of early treatment

Experimental research and clinical experience have shown that pain which is allowed to go on untreated for a long time actually makes the nervous system more sensitive to pain and the patient more prone to experience it. Also, the effect of prolonged pain is to make the treatment of it less effective. So, for these two reasons, it is important for post-herpetic pain to be treated at the earliest possible stage. Patience and stoicism, although admirable, are positively to be discouraged. If you find that, in spite of the healing and disappearance of the rash, the pain of shingles persists, do seek further medical assistance without delay.

Is prevention possible?

A few years ago we used a 40 per cent solution of Idoxuridine in di-methyl-sulphoxide for this purpose. The trade name for this solution is 'Herplex'. Herplex was painted on to the affected area as soon as the rash appeared and it was claimed that, in some cases, this would prevent pain. Idoxuridine (see Chapter 8) certainly had some effect against the VZ virus and the theory was that the shingles attack could be aborted. One hears less about this remedy these days, so perhaps it was not so successful as was originally thought.

Some medical practitioners believe that early shingles should be treated with steroids, so as to prevent the complication of post-herpetic pain. Steroids can certainly minimize inflammation and, to this extent, can be very valuable. But they also interfere markedly with the defensive mechanisms against infection. There is no general approval of this method.

Analgesics

Drugs used to control pain are called 'analgesics'. Aspirin, paracetamol, codeine and morphine are examples of such drugs, but there are many more. The first thing to understand about the use of analgesics is that one should use the mildest drug, in the smallest dosage necessary to relieve the pain, in preference to a stronger drug or a larger dosage. But the pain *must* be relieved and the doctor will, if necessary, employ stronger drugs in order to do so. But he will never use a strong drug like pethidine or a narcotic like morphine if the pain can be removed with a simpler and safer preparation such as, for instance, distalgesic.

Whichever drug is used, it should be used promptly whenever the pain recurs for it has been proved that if doses are spaced so far apart that severe pain is allowed to occur, the effect of the drug is less. In other words, if continuous control is exercised, the necessary dosage will be less than if one waits for the full pain to recur. By using the drug properly one may well, in the end, require a smaller total dosage and achieve a better effect. There is a considerable range of available analgesics and they don't all work in the same way. The fortunate effect of this is that their effect may be additive so that combinations of drugs are often more useful, and capable of controlling pain in smaller dosage, than drugs used singly. So doctors will often prescribe more than one analgesic and ask you to take them together. Sometimes two or more analgesic drugs are combined in the same tablet.

But this principle can be taken further, for the additive effect applies also to different methods of treating pain and I will be describing some of these shortly. The point I want to make, here, is that a very useful effect can be obtained by the judicious combination of analgesics with other treatments, such as physical methods.

The three classes of analgesics

● Probably the most commonly consumed drugs in the world are the mild analgesics, of which aspirin and paracetamol ('Panadol') are typical examples. About two thousands tons of aspirin are swallowed in Britain each year. These drugs may be given in a dose of 600 milligrams every three or four hours, either alone, or in conjunction with other pain-relieving substances. In spite of the popularity of aspirin, paracetamol is probably a rather safer drug. Aspirin can cause bleeding from the lining of the stomach, asthma, urticaria ('nettle-rash'), running at the nose, singing in the ears and even mental confusion, but the more serious effects are uncommon and usually require larger than normal dosage. Panadol in normal dosage such as mentioned above has few side-effects but it is very dangerous to the liver if taken in considerable overdose, so do not increase the dosage.

There are many other mild analgesics, but none are thought to be superior to these two. The combination of analgesics with something to control anxiety, such as a little Valium, can be very useful, and the great majority of people with persistent post-herpetic pain can be effectively relieved in this way without resort to the second group of analgesics.

● The second group consists of drugs which are more powerful, in relieving pain, than the simple analgesics. But they are more liable to induce tolerance so that, over a long period, dosage has to be increased. They are also correspondingly more dangerous than the simpler drugs and have to be used with caution. This group contains drugs such as codeine, pentazocine ('Fortral') and methadone. These are but a few of the many drugs in this group, for one 'wonder drug' after another has been produced each usually being claimed to be more effective and less addictive than anything previously produced. Few, if any, of these claims to non-addictiveness have been sustained. It seems to be a law of nature that a drug with powerful analgesic properties is almost certain to be addictive. Addiction to any of these drugs is certainly possible.

● The third group are the powerful narcotics, such as the opium derivatives, morphine and heroin, and drugs like pethidine. Narcotic drugs are the strongest analgesics. In general, post-herpetic pain does not call for the long-term use of narcotic drugs and no right-thinking doctor will use them if pain can be controlled by simpler means. But, equally, few sympathetic medical men will withhold narcotics if these are the only effective means of relief. It is not *very* uncommon for post-herpetic pain to be so severe that only narcotic drugs will suffice.

The concern, obviously, is about addiction and here one must make a clear distinction between addiction in the sense normally employed, and the tolerance and physical dependence which usually occur in people who have to take narcotics, long-term, for the relief of severe pain. 'Tolerance' just means that the body becomes gradually accustomed to the drug so that progressively larger doses are necessary for the same effect. 'Physical dependence' means that when the drug is no longer necessary, it must be withdrawn gradually if severe symptoms are to be avoided. 'Addiction' really means that the person concerned is now taking the drug for a reason other than the relief of pain and has become psychologically, rather than just physically, dependent on it.

People who are given narcotic drugs *do* sometimes become addicted, but this may be a lesser evil than the continual suffering of pain. Sometimes addiction can be avoided by a change to a different but still effective, non-narcotic drug, while the pain is still occurring. This calls for careful timing and may only be possible if the pain is declining in intensity, so that the alternative drug may be used for a considerable period before treatment can be stopped altogether.

Many people worry that the long-continued use of narcotics will lead to physical deterioration. This worry is largely unfounded. There is a considerable literature describing people who have taken drugs of this class for many years and who, apart from personal and social consequences, seem to have suffered no damage. The undesirable, even tragic, consequences of narcotic indulgence arise from the psychological and moral effects of the need to obtain these drugs illegally, from the criminal activity often required to raise the money to buy them, and from the uncontrolled and often medically dangerous circumstances of their usage.

Narcotic analgesics all produce a tendency to sleepiness and this may call for careful adjustment of dosage or the addition of a 'waking-up' drug, such as amphetamine. But the sleepiness effect of any particular drug varies greatly from one patient to another and it is sometimes possible by trying different narcotics to find one which, in a particular case, has less of this effect than other drugs.

Skin stimulation

Of all the physical methods available for the relief of post-herpetic pain, skin stimulation of the painful area is probably the most generally useful. It is certainly safe. The method is to rub the affected area steadily, and for a prolonged period, with a soft cloth. At first, relief will be obtained only while rubbing, but usually the pain-free period will begin to extend and often quite a long period of relief will follow the rubbing. Sometimes, by intermittent rubbing, it is possible to keep the pain permanently absent. It seems that the continuous passage of low-level nerve impulses caused by the rubbing somehow blocks the pain impulses from getting through. Experts talk about a 'gate' theory of pain, based on a principle similar to that used in the building elements of electronic computers. 'Gates' are electronic switches, through which the passage of a current is permitted, or denied, depending on the presence or absence of a switching signal. Apparently, the small stimulus from skin rubbing provides such a switching signal.

Touch and pressure

Human touch seems to have a special healing significance and here there is obviously a considerable overlap of psychological and physiological effects. There is no doubt that the mere 'laying on of hands' can be of value in the relief of pain, but this seems to be so only if the 'patient' feels that the 'healer' has a genuine hope or expectation of helping. In my own clinical practice, I have noticed that touch can convey to patients a deeper awareness of my concern than any verbal communication, and I am sure that this often increases the effectiveness of my treatment. Studies on the effects of the behaviour of nurses have shown that patients who were not touched considered that their nurses were only concerned to get the job over and done with. I have little doubt that 'faith healing' works, or, at least, confers benefit, in some cases.

So it seems probable that it is the awareness of concern for oneself that makes touch helpful in pain. Certainly, the effect of pain is greatly influenced by the state of mind of the sufferer.

Firm pressure has always been used, almost instinctively, for the relief of pain. Such pressure may be applied with the hand and is most effective if done by a second person. Also, different ways of pressing – either with the flat of the palm, the ball of the thumb, the finger-tips or even with the knuckles – should be tried. I hope the exponents of the ancient Chinese art of acupressure (acupuncture without needles) will forgive me if I refer to the practice in this context. For centuries, acupressure has been used for the relief of pain as well as for many other purposes. Finger-tip pressure is exerted on the formal 'pressure points', either firmly or lightly, as the case demands, to 'unblock' the 'meridians'. Sometimes, the finger-tip is pressed firmly down and then vibrated, in the manner of a violinist.

Massage is also an instinctive reaction and, given by a

concerned person, can be very comforting and may help to relieve pain.

Acupuncture

Acupuncture is being fairly widely used as a physical method of pain control, but the results are variable and it is still not yet clear to what extent the result is due to the 'placebo effect'. However, there is some evidence to suggest that acupunture does have a physiological basis and works by producing in the brain a morphine-like substance. Pharmacologists have now isolated such a substance from the brain and it has been given the name of 'enkephalin'. The matter is still speculative, but that is no reason not to use a relatively safe therapy like acupuncture, should this be found to be effective.

Another theory about the way in which acupuncture works, involves the concept of substances called 'endorphins', morphine-like substances produced within the body as a result of various stimuli. One of the most powerful stimuli to the production of endorphins is fear – everyone knows that in moments of great fear, pain is often not felt at all – and it is possible that the thought of having long needles stuck into one may result in the secretion of these analgesic endorphins.

Acupuncture, for the relief of pain, is being practised increasingly by conventionally trained doctors. It has become an accepted method in many pain clinics, as a supplement to other techniques, and being cheap and safe, is growing in popularity.

Local heat

Local heat has long been regarded as a useful measure for the relief of pain, and a great variety of methods of applying heat has been developed. These range from simple measures, such as hot-water bottles or massage with skin-stimulating liniments such as methyl salicylate (oil of wintergreen), to the most sophisticated microwave or ultra-sonic apparatus. Radiant heat from focused lamps or small electric fires, electric heating pads, hot melted wax, even sun-bathing, can all be helpful in the relief of pain. Should local heat be found helpful, it may be worth trying to arrange for a visit to a physiotherapist for treatment with diathermy or ultrasound. As with several other forms of physical treatment, the hope is that the period of freedom from pain will be sustained for some time after the application of heat.

The cold spray

Some patients find this method very helpful. An aerosol spray of a liquid used in refrigeration, called tri-chloro-fluoro-methane, is sprayed liberally, and repeatedly, over the whole of the painful area until the skin is well cooled. If pain relief is experienced, the method is worth persevering with, the spray being repeated every time the pain returns. This means that spraying will be very frequent at first, but, as with the rubbing technique, the hope is that the interval between treatments and the return of pain will progressively increase. If this does not happen, then the spray method is best abandoned as being uneconomical.

Some people find that eventually they can keep themselves relatively free from pain by only two or three applications a day. Others find a combination of spray and mild analgesics works well. Cold applied in other ways may also be useful. One handy, and cheaper, method is to use a special gel pack, in a plastic bag, which even when left in a freezer will not become solid, but may be moulded to the part to be cooled. Beware of over-cooling!

Unfortunately, some people with post-herpetic pain find that cold applications make the pain worse rather than better.

Transcutaneous electric nerve stimulation

'Transcutaneous' simply means 'through the skin' and the electric currents used are entirely safe. Small, battery-operated packs called 'TENS' units produce a low-level pulsed or alternating current, the frequency and the amplitude of which can be varied to produce the best effects. Wires from the unit connect to small metal plates which are fixed to the skin in whatever position produces the best results. The person being treated feels a tingling or buzzing sensation which may be so strong that underlying muscles begin to twitch. But this is neither desirable nor necessary and the units are normally adjusted until the sensation is only just perceptible.

Many different TENS models have been designed and several types are used in NHS clinics. The electrodes are normally placed on the skin in such a way that they bridge the painful area, but it is sometimes found that placement in different positions is more effective. Some patients, after stimulation for half an hour have enjoyed relief from pain for as long as eight hours. Others have been relieved only for so long as the TENS unit was turned on.

Many patients with post-herpetic pain have found TENS valuable. But, others, after brief initial encouragement, have not. However, failure should not be assumed until various different units have been tried, each with a range of placements of the skin electrodes. Some commercial units are badly designed and ineffective.

Anaesthetic injections

This is a fairly extreme measure and is justified only in cases of severe pain. A long-acting local anaesthetic drug (the most popular is called 'Marcaine' or 'Duracaine') is injected under the skin in the affected area. This will always relieve pain for the duration of the anaesthetic action, which, in the case of Marcaine, is about four hours. But what is hoped for is that the period of relief of pain will extend well beyond the normal time of anaesthesia. This does not often happen, but sometimes there *is* relief for several days. After this, the pain gradually returns and the treatment has to be repeated. The effect of local anaesthetics can sometimes be enhanced by the addition of steroids.

A more radical way of using local anaesthetics is to inject them, not into the skin, but around the trunk of the nerve itself, so as to block the passage of nerve impulses to the brain. This is done using a very long-acting oily preparation of anaesthetic, and cases have been reported where the relief has been permanent. More commonly, the period of useful effect varies from three weeks to three months. The method is not free from disadvantage and it may be difficult to block the sensory nerve without affecting the motor nerve too. Also, as we have seen, complete anaesthesia means that the area of skin supplied by the nerve becomes vulnerable to unnoticed damage. Apart from that, local anaesthesia is unpleasant; some people prefer pain, so long as it is not too severe. In general, nerve block is more suitable for shingles of the trunk than for ophthalmic shingles.

Surgical treatment

This is the most extreme measure of all and should not be considered unless all other possible treatment has failed and the pain is making life intolerable. Actual cutting of the nerves affords some relief of pain, but this may fail as the nerve regenerates.

Post-script

The acute stage of shingles is bearable because it is of limited duration. But when post-herpetic pain occurs, it is helpful to know of the various treatments now available. Obviously, only some of these methods can be adopted without medical assistance but there are now about 200 pain clinics in this country and referral to one of these may be arranged by a GP or by a hospital specialist.

8

Anti-viral Drugs

For years doctors believed that viruses were beyond the reach of antibiotic drugs and that it was unlikely that any would ever be developed which could attack organisms like the VZ virus, in the way that penicillin attacks the streptococcus. But in recent years, exciting new drugs have been developed and the therapeutic barrier which has stood for so long between control of the larger organisms and control of the viruses has been knocked down.

One of the earliest of these drugs, idoxuridine, was developed in 1959. This drug is very useful for surface infections with herpes viruses (it has been used extensively by eye specialists for herpes ulcers of the cornea) but is of limited value for more severe and internal virus infections, mainly because the drug tended to stop human cells from replicating too. This effect was most serious in the rapidly reproducing cells of the bone marrow and the result was a dangerous drop in the output of essential blood and other cells. So idoxuridine was only justified for internal use in severe and life-threatening virus infections.

Another drug which has proved useful but again only for surface application is tri-fluoro-thymidine. More than twenty promising anti-viral drugs have now been produced, almost all of them showing some disadvantage or other, but one drug has put all the others in the shade and promises to be of major value.

Acyclovir

Wellcome agent 248U is the chemical compound 9-(2-Hydroxyethoxymethyl) guanine; 2-Amino-1, 9-dihydro-9-(2-hydroxyethoxymethyl) purin-6-one! The exclamation mark is not part of the formula. This recently developed mouthful has been shown to be highly effective against VZ and herpes simplex viruses and is remarkably safe even when given by injection directly into the bloodstream. For convenience it is called 'acyclovir' and it is the most important advance in virus treatment for twenty-five years. The beauty of it is that it acts specifically on the substance required for DNA virus replication and hardly at all on the equivalent substance required for body cell replication. That means that the drug has very little action (and consequently, danger) except in the presence of viruses.

Acyclovir is extremely effective in preventing replication of both VZ viruses and the very similar herpes simplex viruses that cause venereal herpes, cold sores and eye ulcers. Yet the dose of the drug effective against the viruses is very safe to the patient. Acyclovir is now available in tablet form, as an ophthalmic ointment and skin cream, and as a powder to make up into an intravenous injection.

The Minnesota trial

In June 1983, the prestigious *New England Journal of Medicine* published the results of a trial of acyclovir in patients with shingles. Ninety-four patients, in many different hospitals, were studied and about thirty physicians were involved. All the patients were immunocompromised but none had a life-threatening infection. So far as was possible, they were enrolled into the trial within three days of the first sign of the rash. Each patient gave full consent and it was explained that half of them would receive the active drug and the other half an identical-seeming, but non-active, substitute.

Every detail of their medical histories and of the rash were recorded. Blood and biochemical tests were carried out and samples were taken from the blisters to confirm the shingles diagnosis. A computer allocated the acyclovir in accordance with a random code. Neither the doctors nor the patients knew who was getting the real drug and who the dummy. Only the computer had a record of this. This method is called a 'double-blind' trial, and it is now a standard routine in medical research. It is designed to avoid bias by any participant and to balance the effect on the outcome that might be more due to patients' awareness that they had been treated with a drug, rather than the drug itself. This is known as the 'placebo effect'.)

The acyclovir and the placebo were given by injection into a vein, three times a day for seven days, and all the patients were checked daily for seven days and then repeatedly at slightly longer intervals. At each check, all the tests were repeated and blisters were sampled so as to note when viruses ceased to be produced.

The results clearly showed the efficacy of acyclovir:

● None of the people who were treated with acyclovir, even after the third day, suffered progression of the shingles.

● None developed generalized or neurological shingles.

● The rash and redness cleared more quickly.

● Fewer new blisters were produced.

● The skin healed faster.

● The pain settled faster in the acyclovir group, although in some, it returned after the end of the week's treatment.

The researchers concluded that while a week was probably not long enough to prevent post-herpetic pain, the VZ virus was cleared from the skin vesicles very much more quickly in the acyclovir recipients. The drug was well tolerated and no significant change was caused in the results of the laboratory tests. Its safety seems assured.

It is now generally accepted that acyclovir is the drug of choice in conditions such as herpes virus encephalitis (inflammation of the brain). To quote a leading article in the *British Medical Journal* in January 1985, '. . . acyclovir is sufficiently potent and non-toxic to use in any severe or life-threatening condition caused by herpes simplex viruses 1 and 11 and VZ virus.' So impressive are the results of using this drug, that of the one hundred and seventy-six papers published on VZ virus in major English medical journals between January, 1980 and March, 1985, more dealt with acyclovir than any other single aspect of the subject.

Interferon

Because of the wide range of its action, interferon is believed to be one of the most promising advances in medical treatment since penicillin. It is a powerful, natural substance produced by many cells, especially lymphocytes, and acts by preventing invading viruses from taking cells over. Interferon is highly effective in many virus illnesses including hepatitis, influenza and the common cold (it also acts against those viruses which cause tumours). It is effective in controlling the spread of VZ virus in immunocompromised people and can be life-saving.

Initially it was manufactured by gradual purification of tiny quantities from living cells, but recently it has been found possible to insert the gene that codes for interferon into a bacterium so that when this reproduces,

68

the enormous resulting clones of altered bacteria auto-matically produce large quantities of interferon. This means that greater quantities are becoming available at economic cost and we are likely to hear much more about this remarkable substance.

What about a vaccine?

Can shingles be prevented by vaccination? The 'B' lymphocytes can, and do, produce immunoglobulins to VZ virus and the levels of these immunoglobulins are often quite high in older people who develop shingles. Unfortunately, this indicates the relative uselessness of vaccination against shingles. If the immunoglobulins were able to attack the viruses in the nerve ganglions, we would never get shingles. So, although it is an easy matter to obtain serum from people with zoster immune globulin ('gamma globulin') and although such serum can be used to protect immunocompromised children from the chicken-pox which they so easily acquire and which could be very dangerous to them, it has little or no part to play in the general prevention of shingles.

Glossary

AIDS Acquired immune deficiency syndrome. Shingles occurs in this disease, and partial immune deficiency is important in the causation of shingles.

Antibody A protective protein (immunoglobulin) which attacks 'foreign' material, such as viruses. Antibodies are selected to fit the intruder. People with shingles usually show high levels of antibodies matching VZ virus.

'B' cells The lymphocytes which are selected for their fitness to deal with the invaders. Their cloned descendants, the plasma cells, manufacture the immunoglobulins (antibodies).

Cell-mediated immunity This is vital for the control of shingles; if it declines dormant VZ viruses are able to flare up and cause shingles. The cells concerned are the 'T' lymphocytes.

Chicken-pox Caused by the same virus which causes shingles. The initial infection with VZ virus usually occurs in childhood and causes chicken-pox. Some of the viruses then remain in the body and years later may reactivate to cause shingles.

Clone A line of completely identical cells. Different 'B' cell clones are the sources of specific antibodies against the infections we have had in the past. Most of us have 'B' cell clones which produce antibodies against shingles, but these cannot reach the VZ viruses which are actually within nerve cells.

Cold sores   Mouth blisters causes by the herpes simplex virus, which is almost identical to the VZ virus.

Cornea   The front lens of the eye. It can be involved in ophthalmic shingles.

Cortisol   This is the natural steroid hormone produced by the adrenal glands in response to stress. It helps us to cope with the stress, but may also interfere with cell-mediated immunity – and this is probably why shingles is often precipitated by stress.

Cow-pox   A disease caused by a modified smallpox virus, successfully used by Jenner to vaccinate against smallpox. This was the first major step towards our present understanding of conditions like shingles and of their control.

Cranial nerves   These are pairs of nerves emerging directly from the brain. The fifth nerve, the trigeminal, is involved in ophthalmic shingles.

Cytotoxic drugs   These are used in the treatment of cancer and other serious conditions. People taking these are prone to shingles.

DNA   Deoxy-ribo-nucleic acid. The genetic material found in all cells. DNA is the master-plan, written in genes, which determines all the characteristics of the cell's descendants. VZ viruses consist almost entirely of DNA.

Encephalitis   Inflammation of the brain. Can be caused by VZ or herpes simplex viruses, in immunocompromised people, but this is a rare occurrence.

Ganglion   A collection of nerve-cell bodies in which the shingles (VZ) viruses lurk for years. On becoming active again, they produce a severe ganglionitis (inflammation of the ganglion) which is the major element in shingles.

Glaucoma   A condition of raised pressure within the eye which *may* occur in ophthalmic shingles.

Grafts   Tissue grafts, from a donor, will be rejected if the body's immune system is functioning. So for successful kidney or heart transplants the immune system is deliberately, medically knocked out. But the loss of immunity means that the patient becomes more prone to conditions like shingles.

Hemianopia   Loss of half the field of vision. A rare complication of generalized shingles. Recovery is usual.

Hemiplegia   Paralysis of one side of the body. *May* occur in shingles encephalitis. Common from arterial disease but rare in shingles.

Herpes   The name commonly applied to an infection with herpes simplex virus: 'cold sores' or venereal herpes. Has much in common with shingles. The word 'herpes' literally means 'creeping' and indeed, the rash does creep along.

Herpes zoster   This is the medical name for shingles. 'HZ' virus is an abbreviation of 'herpes zoster' virus.

Hyperaesthesia   The state of excessive sensitivity of the skin which occurs in the affected area prior to the appearance of the shingles rash. This sensitivity is also a common characteristic of post-herpetic pain.

Immune deficiency   A reduction in the efficiency of the immunological protective systems of the body. May be due to a deficiency of 'B' or 'T' cells, or both. May be congenital (present at birth) or acquired. May be the result of medical treatment.

Immunocompromised   Liable to the ill-effects of immune deficiency.

Immunoglobulins Antibodies. Protective protein substances produced by the plasma cell clones of 'B' lymphocytes.

Interferon A naturally occurring substance which has a powerful anti-viral and anti-cancer action. Will be extremely important in medicine, in the future.

Lyphocytes Small, round, white cells. Found in the blood and, in vast numbers, in the lymph glands. They consist of two main types – 'B' cells and 'T' cells – and are the basis of immunity.

Motor nerves Nerves which carry impulses from the brain or spinal cord to the muscles. Much less commonly affected in shingles, than sensory nerves.

Nerve cell This consists of the cell body, which contains the nucleus, and a very long nerve fibre connecting it with the central nervous system. In shingles, VZ viruses invade the cell body.

Ophthalmic Relating to the eye.

Ophthalmic herpes zoster Shingles affecting the sensory nerve to the eye, the trigeminal nerve. This nerve also supplies the skin of the upper lid and forehead, so this is where the rash appears.

Plasma cells These are the cloned offspring of 'B' cells and produce immunoglobulins (antibodies).

Sensory nerve A nerve subserving all forms of sensation and carry impulses from the skin and body generally, to the brain. Shingles is primarily an infection of sensory nerves.

Spinal cord The downward extension from the brain, carrying nerve pathways to and from the body. Can be affected by shingles.

Stress   Believed to be an important precipitating factor in shingles, because stress causes the body to produce the hormone Cortisol and this interferes with cell-mediated immunity.

'T' cells   The lymphocytes which protect against foreign invading material especially that which alters cells. Active against our own body cells which have been invaded by viruses or those which have become cancerous.

Thymus   The neck organ where the 'T' cells are matured; consequently they are called 'T' cells.

Trigeminal nerve   The fifth cranial nerve. It has three branches, of which the upper ('ophthalmic') branch is affected in ophthalmic shingles.

Uveitis   Inflammation of the iris and the focusing muscle of the eye. Can occur in ophthalmic herpes zoster.

Vaccination   The use of a safely modified germ or virus to persuade the immune system to produce protective antibodies. Not much use in shingles, unfortunately, although a vaccine does exist which is valuable for very young, unprotected children threatened by chicken-pox.

Varicella   The medical name for chicken-pox. Varicella-zoster is the name of the virus which causes both chicken-pox and shingles.

Vesicles   The small blisters occurring in the rashes of shingles and chickenpox. These blisters teem with VZ viruses.

Virus   An infecting organism, much too small to be

seen with even the most powerful conventional microscope. This organism can survive and reproduce only within a host cell.

VZ virus   The varicella-zoster virus.

Index

Also published by Sheldon Press

Coping with Depression and Elation

Dr PATRICK McKEON

Everyone who suffers from depression and mood swings will find this book invaluable. It describes simply and sympathetically the known causes, symptoms and treatment of depressive moods. The author tells us why we experience 'ups and downs', discusses fully how to recognise mood swings, and reveals the problems that can occur if a true depressive illness is not diagnosed and treatment given. He describes how depression and elation are successfully treated today and gives advice on how both sufferers and their families can cope with a depressive mood illness.

If you suffer from this problem, Dr McKeon shows that there is no need to feel overwhelmed by it; the vast majority of us can come to terms with it and lead happy and fulfilled lives.

ISBN 0 85969 502 6   **£7·95 cased**
        0 85969 503 4   **£3·95 paper**

Fight Your Phobia – and Win

DAVID LEWIS

Do you fear enclosed spaces? Are you afraid of snakes, spiders or cats? Or perhaps you are frightened of venturing out of your home? Do certain kinds of people, situations, objects or activities make you feel very nervous for no sensible reason?

If you feel great anxiety about things that other people seem to take for granted, you may be suffering from a phobia. This is not unusual, and not something to be ashamed of. All phobias, no matter how apparently impossible to deal with, can be successfully overcome. This book shows you how.

David Lewis, a practising psychologist, describes how phobias develop, and explains how they can be conquered by using a practical, simple and proven technique. You need never feel afraid again.

ISBN 0 85969 405 4   **£6·95 cased**
        0 85969 498 8   **£3·95 paper**

An A–Z of Alternative Medicine

B. HAFEN and K. FRANDSEN

Does acupuncture cure headaches? Will hypnosis help you to stop smoking? What are herbal medicines used for? Can yoga ease backache?

These, and many other questions, are answered in this informative and objective guide on today's most popular alternative healing methods. Alphabetically arranged for easy reference, it includes biofeedback, biorhythms, dance therapy, faith healing, massage and meditation, to name only a few of the topics covered. Each technique is clearly and simply described by the authors. They also describe the background to the different methods and explain how each one is used.

You may be interested in improving your health by alternative healing, or you may just wish to learn more about the subject. In either case, *An A–Z of Alternative Medicine* can provide you with the plain facts about a whole range of alternative treatments.

ISBN 0 85969 427 5   **£6·95 cased**
      0 85969 428 3   **£3·95 paper**

Body Language

ALLAN PEASE

What people say to you is often very different from what they think or feel.

Now with *Body Language* you can correctly interpret other people's thoughts by their gestures. Allan Pease is *the* international expert on body language – communicating without words.

Body Language is fun to read and will quickly teach you:

★ How to tell if someone is lying
★ How to make yourself more likeable
★ How to get co-operation from other people
★ How to successfully conduct interviews and business negotiations
★ How to pick a suitable partner

Buy it and try it. Today.

ISBN 0 85969 407 0   **£7·95 cased**
      0 85969 406 2   **£2·95 paper**

Women and Depression
A practical self-help guide

DEIDRE SANDERS

Every year one in five women takes tranquillizers for depression. Many more of us try to cope without consulting a doctor – often because we feel it should be possible to control such 'negative' feelings without professional help.

This positive and practical book will help you and your family to understand what may have triggered your depression, and how it can be overcome. It describes the common causes of depression, such as pre-menstrual tension, a broken marriage, childbirth, the menopause, bereavement, loneliness and many others. It tells you what symptoms you should look out for, what should be done, the different treatments prescribed and, most important of all, how you can help yourself.

If you feel 'low', *Women and Depression* will give you the guidance and sympathetic advice that you need.

ISBN 0 85969 418 6   **£6·95 cased**
      0 85969 419 4   **£2·50 paper**

Loneliness

Why it happens and how to overcome it

Dr TONY LAKE

Nearly all of us feel lonely at some time and many of us feel lonely most of the time. You may have felt lonely as long as you can remember and expect to go on for the rest of your life in this way. Or you may suffer from acute loneliness which you know will end in a matter of weeks or months. You can be lonely whatever the circumstances, whether you are living alone or surrounded by people. None of us is immune, all ages are affected – children, teenagers, young men and women, the middle-aged, and the elderly.

There are two ways to deal with loneliness, and both ways depend on you. One way is to cope with it, that is to live through it and to carry on despite the painful nature of the feeling, and this book is partly about ways to cope. The second way is to overcome it so that it never has the same power to hurt you again, and the rest of the book will help in your search for a more permanent solution.

ISBN 0 85969 285 X   **£2·50**

Meeting People is Fun

How to overcome shyness

Dr PHYLLIS M. SHAW

Do you stay home alone on Saturday nights because you're too shy to accept a party invitation or walk into a pub? Would you really like to ask your neighbours in for tea but are afraid they'd say no? Feeling shy can stop you enjoying life and make you very lonely.

We often feel shy when mixing with people because we are frightened they won't like us or that we will make fools of ourselves, *Meeting People is Fun* explains these all too common fears and gives sound advice about coping with potentially terrifying situations.

As your confidence increases you'll be able to walk into a roomful of strangers. And you'll know what to say after you've said hello!

ISBN 0 85969 136 5   **£2·50 paper**